COMPLETE GUIDE TO ADENOIDECTOMY

Comprehensive Surgery Techniques, Recovery Tips, And Post-Operative Care For Adults And Children, Expert Advice On Risks, Benefits, And Complications Management

DR. BRUNO HORAN

Copyright © 2023 by Dr. Bruno Horan

All rights reserved. Except for brief quotations embodied in critical reviews and certain other noncommercial uses permitted by copyright law, no part of this publication may be reproduced, distributed, or transmitted in any form or by any means, Including photocopying, recording, or other electronic or mechanical methods, without the prior written permission of the publisher.

Disclaimer:

The information provided in this book, is intended for general informational purposes only and should not be considered as professional advice.

The author has made every effort to ensure the accuracy of the information presented. However, readers are advised to consult with a qualified healthcare professional before attempting any herbal remedies or making significant changes to their wellness routine. Individual health conditions vary, and what may be suitable for one person may not be appropriate for another.

It is important to note that the author is not in any endorsement deal, partnership, or affiliation with any organization, brand, or company mentioned in this book. Any references to specific products or services are based on the author's personal experience or general knowledge and do not imply an endorsement or promotion of those products or services

Contents

CHAPTER ONE 11
  ADEOIDS' ANATOMY AND FUNCTION 11
    Anatomy Of The Adenoids In Detail 11
    Function Within The Immune System 12
    The Transition Of Adenoids From Childhood To Adulthood 13
    Typical Issues Related To Adenoids 14

CHAPTER TWO 17
  ADENOID PROBLEM DIAGNOSIS 17
    Adenoid Enlargement Symptoms 17
    Tools And Techniques For Diagnosis 18
    Comprehending Diagnostic Test Outcomes 19
    Case Studies Of Typical Diagnostic Circumstances 21
    The Value Of Prompt Identification And Intervention 22

CHAPTER THREE 25
  SIGNS AND SYMPTOMS OF ADENOIDECTOMY 25
    Conditions That Call For An Adenoidectomy 26

Distinguishing Adenoidectomy From Other Therapies 27

Evaluating The Benefits Vs. Risks Of Surgery 28

Case Studies Of Patients And Indications 29

Medical Association Guidelines 30

CHAPTER FOUR 33

GETTING READY FOR SURGERY 33

Preoperative Medical Assessments And Exams ...33

Guidelines For Patients And Their Caregivers...... 34

Controlling Your Expectations And Anxiety 36

Required Records And Consent Forms 37

Working Along With The Surgical Team 38

CHAPTER FIVE 41

THE PROCEDURE FOR ADENOIDECTOMY 41

Detailed Account Of The Surgical Procedure:...... 41

Options And Considerations For Anesthesia:....... 42

Instruments And Surgical Methods Used: 43

Monitoring During Surgery And Safety Procedures: 46

CHAPTER SIX 49

LONG-TERM HEALTH AND SUPPORT 49

Recheck Appointments And Expectations 50

Things Not To Do While Recovering 51

Dietary Guidelines Following Surgery 52

Recognizing And Handling Any Postponed Issues 53

CHAPTER SEVEN 55

COMMON ISSUES AND DIFFICULTIES 55

Handling Typical Postoperative Problems 56

Identifying Infection Or Complication Signs 57

Resolving The Concerns Of Parents And Caregivers 58

Techniques For A Quick And Problem-Free Recuperation 59

CHAPTER EIGHT 61

DETAILED FAQS 61

Frequently Asked Questions About Adenoidectomy Addressed 63

Testimonials And Experiences From Patients 65

CONCERNING THIS BOOK

The book "Adenoidectomy" provides a thorough overview of the complexities of adenoid surgery, providing insightful information to patients and medical experts alike. It starts with a thorough examination of the morphology and immunological importance of adenoids, emphasizing their development from childhood to adulthood and their vital role in the immune system. This basic knowledge lays the groundwork for more in-depth talks later in the book by helping readers comprehend the range of problems that can occur with adenoids, including their relationship to other ENT difficulties.

An important part that helps to clarify the process of determining adenoid-related concerns is diagnosing adenoid disorders. It discusses the signs and symptoms of adenoid enlargement and goes into detail on the diagnostic techniques and equipment, like endoscopy and X-rays, that are used to find these issues. Through the use of case examples and a focus on the significance of early detection and intervention, the book provides readers with the necessary tools to identify and swiftly address adenoid difficulties, which is essential for successful treatment.

The book also goes into great detail on the problems that call for an adenoidectomy and what qualifies as an indication for the procedure. It helps readers understand when surgery is the best option by differentiating adenoidectomy from other therapies. A comprehensive viewpoint on weighing the advantages and disadvantages of adenoidectomy is provided in this part, which is enhanced by patient case studies and recommendations from medical groups.

The process of getting ready for surgery is explained in detail, including the preoperative assessments, guidelines for patients and caregivers, and techniques for controlling expectations and anxiety. By doing this, it is made sure that patients and their families are ready for surgery. The book is a priceless tool for learning the specifics of the surgical operation since it offers a detailed account of the adenoidectomy process, complete with anesthetic choices, surgical methods, and intraoperative safety precautions.

Postoperative care is as comprehensive and includes rapid recovery room protocols, pain management, nourishment, hydration, and complications monitoring. It provides helpful home care advice and discharge guidelines to help ensure a speedy recovery. By providing patients with a comprehensive post-surgery roadmap, follow-up appointment schedules, and dietary suggestions, the long-term recovery and care section goes above and beyond in providing support.

The book addresses frequent worries and complications and offers advice on how to handle postoperative problems including fevers and sore throats, spot infection symptoms, and know when to see a physician. Concerns from parents and other caregivers are also covered, along with tips for a quick recovery devoid of complications. By addressing frequently asked concerns, dispelling falsehoods, and providing patient stories and testimonials, the comprehensive FAQs section enhances the reader's comprehension even more. For medical professionals, patients, and their families, or everyone else engaged in the adenoidectomy process, this book is a vital resource.

CHAPTER ONE

ADEOIDS' ANATOMY AND FUNCTION

Anatomy Of The Adenoids In Detail

The pharyngeal tonsils, or adenoids, are a mass of lymphoid tissue situated behind the nasal cavity in the upper region of the throat. Adenoids are located behind the nasal passages and slightly above the roof of the mouth, high on the posterior wall of the nasopharynx. The palatine tonsils can be seen via the mouth, while adenoids are difficult to see without special tools. Like other tonsillar tissues, they are made of lymphatic tissue and have a thin layer of epithelium covering them.

The glossopharyngeal and vagus nerve branches innervate the adenoids, which have an abundant supply of blood vessels. Due to their function in the immune response and the possibility of causing symptoms when swollen or infected, this vascular and nerve supply is crucial.

Function Within The Immune System

Adenoids are important for the immune system, especially in the early years of life. They are a component of the body's initial defense system against infections that enter through the mouth and nose.

Immune cells like lymphocytes, which are found in adenoids, are in charge of recognizing and warding off infectious pathogens. To stop bacteria and viruses from spreading to other areas of the body, these immune cells absorb and digest them.

Adenoids are quite active throughout the first few years of life and play a major role in the immune system's development. They aid in the generation of antibodies and in teaching the immune system how to identify and react to infections. However, the adenoids become less important and usually get smaller as a person ages and their immune system develops.

The Transition Of Adenoids From Childhood To Adulthood

Childhood is when adenoids are most prevalent, especially between the ages of three and seven. They participate actively in the immune response at this time, and recurrent exposure to infections may occasionally cause them to expand. This expansion may result in several symptoms and issues.

Children's immune systems become more effective as they age, and their adenoids gradually recede. The adenoids sometimes undergo a considerable size reduction by adolescence, and in certain adults, they may even nearly totally atrophy.

Because of this natural retreat, problems associated with adolescence become less frequent as people age.

Adenoids, however, can occasionally linger and create issues well into adulthood.

Typical Issues Related To Adenoids

Adenoids that are enlarged can cause several health problems, especially in young people. Obstructive sleep apnea (OSA), in which the enlarged adenoids restrict the airway during sleep, is one of the most prevalent issues.

This results in breathing difficulties and frequent awakenings. OSA is characterized by snoring, restless sleep, and weariness during the day.

The recurring infection is another prevalent problem. Increased adenoids may serve as a breeding ground for bacteria and viruses, which can cause recurrent episodes of sinusitis, otitis media (ear infections), and sore throats. Nasal congestion, postnasal drip, and chronic cough are examples of symptoms that might continue after a chronic infection.

Sometimes, enlarged adenoids can obstruct the Eustachian tubes, which go from the middle ear to the nasopharynx, causing problems with proper ear function. This may result in an accumulation of fluid in the middle ear, which raises the risk of ear infections and causes hearing loss.

The Connection Between Other ENT Problems and Adenoids

Numerous ear, nose, and throat (ENT) conditions are intimately associated with adenoids. For example, the Eustachian tubes flow into the nasopharynx close to the adenoids and aid in controlling air pressure and draining fluid from the middle ear. These tubes may become blocked by enlarged adenoids, which can result in middle ear infections and hearing issues.

The sinuses may also be impacted by long-term nasal congestion brought on by swollen adenoids. Normal sinus drainage is hampered by blocked nasal passages, and this can result in sinus infections and chronic sinusitis. Furthermore, children who mouth breathe owing to nasal obstruction may experience alterations in their face growth, dental problems, and dry mouth.

Recognizing and treating linked ENT diseases requires an understanding of the anatomy, function, and potential difficulties related to the adenoids. Efficient handling and therapy have the potential to reduce indications and enhance general well-being, especially in kids who are most frequently impacted by issues associated with adenoids.

CHAPTER TWO

ADENOID PROBLEM DIAGNOSIS

Adenoid Enlargement Symptoms

A common illness in children, adenoid hypertrophy can present with a variety of symptoms. Chronic nasal congestion is one of the most prevalent signs. Children who have enlarged adenoids may often breathe through their lips due to obstructions in their nasal passages. During sleep, this mouth breathing may be accompanied by snoring and a voice that sounds nasal. Recurrent ear infections are another important symptom to consider. The blockage of the Eustachian tubes by enlarged adenoids can result in fluid accumulation and subsequent infections.

Sleep apnea, difficulty swallowing, and restless sleep are other symptoms. Parents may observe that their child's breathing pauses frequently while they sleep, which may lead to the youngster waking up a lot and feeling exhausted during the day. Children may also have symptoms like foul breath, runny nose, and persistent cough. These symptoms should be regularly monitored because they can have a serious negative effect on a child's general health and quality of life.

Tools And Techniques For Diagnosis

Various diagnostic tools and approaches are used by healthcare providers to accurately diagnose adenoid disorders. A physical examination is one of the main approaches. During this examination, the physician will examine the back of the throat and ears to search for indications of infection or adenoidal growth.

Another useful method for identifying adenoid problems is an X-ray. The size and shape of the adenoids can be seen on a lateral neck X-ray, which can assist the physician assess whether or not they are enlarged. This non-invasive imaging method clearly shows adenoid hypertrophy.

A more direct diagnostic technique is endoscopy. It entails examining the adenoids and adjacent structures with an endoscope, a flexible tube equipped with a light, and a camera.

The doctor can see the size of the adenoids and any potential blockages they may be causing with this surgery, which is frequently performed under topical anesthetic.

Nasal endoscopy can also assist in determining whether any further sinus or nasal problems are causing the symptoms.

Comprehending Diagnostic Test Outcomes

Determining the best course of action for adenoid disorders requires interpreting the results of diagnostic examinations.

An enlarged adenoid will show up as a mass blocking the airway on an X-ray. Doctors can determine the need for surgery, such as an adenoidectomy, based on the extent of obstruction.

The results of an endoscopy give a more thorough picture. The precise size of the adenoids and their effect on other structures, such as the nasal passageways and Eustachian tubes, can be seen in the endoscopic images.

It could be advised to have surgery if it is discovered that the adenoids are noticeably enlarged, resulting in a major obstruction or infection.

Along with these diagnostic findings, doctors also take the patient's symptoms into account. For example, the probability of recommending an adenoidectomy increases if a kid has a history of recurrent ear infections or major breathing issues and the diagnostic tests show that the child has adenoid hypertrophy.

Case Studies Of Typical Diagnostic Circumstances

Case studies offer useful information about how to diagnose adenoid issues. An initial physical examination might be performed on a seven-year-old child who presents with chronic nasal congestion and frequent ear infections, for instance. A lateral neck X-ray is ordered by the doctor, who suspects swollen adenoids; the results demonstrate considerable adenoid hypertrophy.

The results are confirmed by an endoscopy, which shows that the adenoids are obstructing the Eustachian tubes. In light of the persistent infections and respiratory issues, the physician suggests an adenoidectomy.

In another case, a physical examination raises concerns for a five-year-old child who has persistent sleep apnea and restless sleep, so the child gets an endoscopic examination.

The airway is severely obstructed during sleep due to the mild expansion of the adenoids, as revealed by the endoscopy.

To enhance the child's general health and quality of sleep, an adenoidectomy is recommended based on these findings and the severity of the symptoms.

The Value Of Prompt Identification And Intervention

To avoid difficulties and enhance quality of life, it is essential to identify and treat adenoid disorders as soon as possible.

Early detection of adenoid hypertrophy can aid in the successful management of symptoms before they worsen and cause persistent ear infections, obstructive sleep apnea, or serious breathing difficulties.

Early treatment can reduce these symptoms and save long-term health issues; this is frequently done with an adenoidectomy.

By keeping an eye on symptoms and seeking medical attention when they observe chronic problems like nasal congestion, snoring, or mouth breathing, parents and caregivers can play a critical role in early detection. Frequent visits to the pediatrician can also aid in the early detection of adenoid issues, facilitating prompt and efficient treatment.

CHAPTER THREE
SIGNS AND SYMPTOMS OF ADENOIDECTOMY

Adenoids are surgically removed during an adenoidectomy, usually as a result of persistent problems that impair breathing, sleep, or general health. Recurrent infections are one of the main reasons for this operation. Adenoidectomy is generally beneficial for children with persistent ear infections or recurrent episodes of adenoiditis. These infections may result in an ongoing accumulation of fluid in the middle ear, which may cause developmental delays and hearing loss.

Another noteworthy indicator is the presence of obstructive sleep apnea (OSA). Larger adenoids may obstruct the airway as you sleep, leading to breathing pauses and snoring. Behavior issues, low academic performance, and daytime tiredness can all result from this illness. Adenoidectomy is frequently necessary for children with OSA who do not respond to other therapies to restore regular breathing patterns during sleep.

Conditions That Call For An Adenoidectomy

Adenoidectomy is especially required for several medical issues. One such illness is chronic rhinosinusitis, which is characterized by persistent sinus infection and inflammation. By enhancing sinus outflow, excision of the adenoids can help reduce symptoms when medicine and other non-surgical therapies are ineffective.

Otitis medium with effusion (OME) is another condition in which there is persistent fluid in the middle ear without any indication of an acute infection. This may impact the development of speech and language and cause hearing issues. Adenoidectomies, frequently in conjunction with ear tube placement, can enhance auditory function and lessen the likelihood that OME will return.

In addition, anomalies in facial growth and dental problems might result from prolonged mouth breathing and nasal blockage caused by swollen adenoids. Adenoidectomy can help in these situations by opening up the nasal airways and facilitating healthy tooth and face development.

Distinguishing Adenoidectomy From Other Therapies

Adenoidectomy is frequently contrasted with other therapies, such as drugs or less invasive operations. When treating infections and inflammations of the adenoids, medications such as decongestants, nasal steroids, and antibiotics are usually the first to be used.

These therapies, however, might only offer momentary respite and are inappropriate for persistent or recurrent illnesses.

While non-surgical methods such as nasal irrigation may aid in symptom management, they may not tackle the root cause of swollen or persistently infected adenoids.

By eliminating the troublesome tissue, however, an adenoidectomy provides a more permanent cure by lowering the incidence and severity of infections and blockages.

Evaluating The Benefits Vs. Risks Of Surgery

It is important to examine both the possible dangers and benefits of adenoidectomy. Better breathing, lower infection rates, and an overall higher quality of life are frequently the advantages.

This can benefit kids by reducing absences from school, improving sleep quality, and promoting healthy growth and development.

There are hazards associated with every procedure, though. These can include anesthesia-related problems, bleeding, and infections. There may also be postoperative pain and transient swallowing or vocal abnormalities. To ensure that patients and their families have reasonable expectations and are fully informed, healthcare providers should have a thorough discussion about these risks with them.

Case Studies Of Patients And Indications

Analyzing patient case studies can yield important information on when an adenoidectomy is appropriate. For example, when antibiotics and other treatments fail to relieve a six-year-old child's chronic nasal congestion and recurrent ear infections, the youngster may have an adenoidectomy. The child had better hearing and fewer infections after surgery.

In a different instance, an adenoidectomy may be suggested for an eight-year-old child with severe obstructive sleep apnea if sleep testing verifies that swollen adenoids are the main source of airway obstruction.

After surgery, the child's academic achievement, behavior throughout the day, and quality of sleep may all show notable improvements.

Medical Association Guidelines

The use of guidelines from medical groups is crucial in establishing the appropriateness of adenoidectomy. For instance, the American Academy of Otolaryngology-Head and Neck Surgery specifies some requirements for proposing an adenoidectomy, such as the existence of persistent infections that are not alleviated by medication or a severe breathing issue during sleep.

By standardizing care, these recommendations guarantee that patients receive therapies that are supported by evidence.

Additionally, they stress the significance of providing tailored care that takes into consideration each patient's particular needs and circumstances. Following these recommendations enables healthcare professionals to make well-informed decisions that improve patient outcomes.

CHAPTER FOUR

GETTING READY FOR SURGERY

Preoperative Medical Assessments And Exams

To make sure the patient is suitable for surgery, extensive medical examinations and assessments must be completed before an adenoidectomy. A thorough review of the patient's medical history, a physical examination, and sometimes certain diagnostic procedures like blood work, X-rays, or an electrocardiogram (ECG) are all part of these assessments.

These evaluations are meant to reveal any underlying medical issues that might make surgery or the healing process more difficult.

The healthcare professional will inquire about past surgeries, chronic illnesses, allergies, and current medications during the evaluation of medical history. The surgical team can better adjust the anesthesia and surgical strategy to the individual needs of the patient with the use of this information. In addition to focusing on the ears, nose, and throat, the physical examination may also involve a general health assessment to make sure no other issues need to be addressed before surgery.

To obtain a more comprehensive understanding of the patient's general health, diagnostic tests may be prescribed. An ECG can identify any cardiac difficulties, while blood tests can identify possible concerns including anemia or clotting disorders. These assessments are essential to reducing surgical risks and guaranteeing a speedy recovery.

Guidelines For Patients And Their Caregivers

Patients and their caregivers receive comprehensive instructions on how to be ready for surgery on the day of the procedure. Typically, these instructions include advice on fasting before the treatment, which is abstaining from food and liquids after midnight the night before the procedure. To lower the danger of aspiration under anesthesia, fasting is essential.

Also, patients could be given detailed instructions regarding their drugs. Certain drugs may still need to be taken with a tiny sip of water the morning of the procedure, while others may need to be stopped a few days prior. To prevent problems, you must adhere to these directions exactly.

Advice is given to caregivers on how to assist the patient before and following surgery. Since patients won't be able to drive themselves home, this also entails making arrangements for transportation to and from the surgery center.

In addition, caregivers need to be ready to assist with postoperative care, which includes keeping an eye out for any indications of difficulties, making sure the patient gets enough sleep, and administering any recommended medicine.

Controlling Your Expectations And Anxiety

Anxiety around surgery can affect individuals as well as their families. To guarantee a more seamless experience, it's critical to deal with these issues early on. It is important to encourage patients to voice their concerns and ask inquiries. A clear understanding of what to expect will greatly minimize worry.

Healthcare professionals frequently talk about the specifics of the operation, what happens during anesthesia, and the recuperation period. Videos or other visual aids can be useful in clarifying the surgical procedures. Reassurance can be gained from knowing that the technique is standard and from being aware of its advantages.

Caretakers may need to explain adenoidectomy procedures to youngsters in an age-appropriate manner. Books, movies, or even role-playing games might assist kids in comprehending what transpires.

Another way to offer comfort is to bring a blanket or favorite toy with you to the hospital.

Required Records And Consent Forms

A vital step in the preoperative procedure is filling out the consent forms and related paperwork. These records guarantee that the patient has been fully educated about the procedure, is aware of the advantages and dangers, and has been permitted to have the surgery.

Information on the procedure, anesthetic, possible hazards, and anticipated results are usually included in consent forms.

This paperwork must be thoroughly reviewed and signed by the patients or their legal guardians. It's also a chance to clear up any lingering queries or concerns you may have with the healthcare professional.

Identification, insurance information, and medical records are possible additional required documents. To prevent misunderstanding at the last minute, it is advisable to arrange all of this paperwork beforehand. Making use of a checklist can help guarantee that nothing is overlooked.

Working Along With The Surgical Team

A seamless surgical experience requires efficient collaboration with the surgical team. This entails speaking with the anesthesiologist, nurse staff, and surgeon. To confirm arrangements and handle any last-minute concerns, preoperative meetings or calls are frequently organized.

On where and when to arrive at the surgery facility, detailed information will be given by the surgical team.

They will also talk about how long the procedure should take and how long it will take to recover. To guarantee prompt and effective service, it is crucial that you carefully follow these directions.

The surgical team will verify the procedure, go over the patient's medical history, and address any last-minute concerns on the day of the treatment. Additionally, they will confirm that any preoperative guidelines—such as fasting—have been adhered to. This meticulous synchronization guarantees that all parties are in agreement and that the procedure goes without any issues.

CHAPTER FIVE

THE PROCEDURE FOR ADENOIDECTOMY

Detailed Account Of The Surgical Procedure:

The goal of an adenoidectomy is to remove the glands that are positioned at the rear of the nasal canal, known as adenoids.

Breathing problems, recurring ear infections, and other health problems can result from swollen or diseased glands.

To guarantee the patient's comfort and safety during the process, general anesthesia is usually administered before the treatment starts.

After the patient is sedated, the surgeon will gently open the nostrils with a nasal speculum, a specialized tool that allows for improved access to the adenoids. Subsequently, the adenoid tissue at the back of the nose is carefully removed using a small suction instrument or curette. Until all of the troublesome tissue has been removed, this process is repeated.

Any bleeding that occurs after the adenoids are removed is carefully managed with methods like cauterization or packing the area with materials that dissolve.

Finally, before closing the incision and finishing the treatment, the surgeon will make sure the nasal passageways are clear.

Options And Considerations For Anesthesia:

Any surgical treatment, including adenoidectomy, must include anesthesia. General anesthesia is usually administered to patients having adenoidectomy procedures, rendering them fully asleep and unresponsive throughout the procedure. This guarantees them no pain or discomfort and permits the surgical team to do their duties safely and efficiently.

General anesthesia may, however, occasionally be supplemented or substituted with local anesthetic or sedation. This choice is based on the intricacy of the procedure as well as the patient's age, general health, and preferences.

The anesthesia team will go over the risks and benefits of each choice with the patient and perform a complete evaluation of the patient's medical history before the treatment.

Throughout the procedure, they will also keep a careful eye on the patient to make sure they stay comfortable and stable.

Instruments And Surgical Methods Used:

Depending on the patient's demands and the surgeon's preferences, a variety of methods and instruments may be employed during an adenoidectomy. Nevertheless, whether the method is employed, the fundamental steps in the process are always the same.

One popular method is to scrape the adenoid tissue off the back of the nose using a curette, a tiny, spoon-shaped tool.

A more delicate method of removing the tissue is to use a suction device. Certain surgeries may require the use of endoscopic procedures or specialized tools to increase visibility and accuracy.

The surgery aims to remove all of the adenoid tissue with as little damage as possible to the surrounding structures, regardless of the method employed. This guarantees a quicker recovery for the patient and lowers the possibility of complications.

Phases and length of the operation:

The size of the adenoids, the patient's age, and any underlying medical issues can all affect how long an adenoidectomy takes.

On the other hand, the majority of adenoidectomies can be finished in 30 to 45 minutes.

The process usually involves multiple stages, such as administering an anesthetic, placing the patient, setting up the surgical site, extracting the adenoid tissue, and closing the incision.

The surgical team works meticulously and methodically to provide the best possible outcome for the patient at every stage.

Following surgery, the patient is brought to a recovery area to be closely observed while they come out of anesthesia.

 After patients are stable and completely awake, they could be sent home with instructions for follow-up and postoperative care.

Monitoring During Surgery And Safety Procedures:

Many precautions are taken during an adenoidectomy to keep an eye on the patient's vital signs and guarantee their safety at all times. This entails constant observation of vital signs such as blood pressure, oxygen saturation, and heart rate.

The surgical team is trained to identify and act upon any indications of problems or distress in addition to monitoring equipment.

This could entail modifying the anesthetic dosage, offering more assistance with the patient's airway, or doing other suitable measures to preserve their health.

Strict safety procedures are also adhered to to reduce the possibility of infection and other issues during the procedure.

This entails keeping the operating room clean, utilizing sterile tools and supplies, and adhering to predetermined standards for surgical technique and aftercare.

All things considered, adenoidectomy is a safe and efficient treatment for patients of all ages thanks to these intraoperative monitoring and safety measures. The surgical team can minimize risk while achieving ideal results by employing suitable surgical procedures, continuously monitoring the patient during the procedure, and carefully managing the anesthetic.

CHAPTER SIX

LONG-TERM HEALTH AND SUPPORT

The road to recovery following an adenoidectomy is usually simple, but to guarantee a seamless healing procedure, it's critical to comprehend the long-term care and recovery process. Although each person's recuperation process may differ slightly, there are some standard protocols to adhere to.

Normal Timetable for Recuperation

Following an adenoidectomy, patients may feel some discomfort, including congestion and sore throats. But they are usually only temporary symptoms that go away in a few days. To give your body time to heal after surgery, make sure you get enough rest and limit your physical activity during the first week.

Many patients start to experience noticeable improvements in their symptoms by the end of the first week, including better breathing and less nasal congestion. But it could take a few weeks for a full recovery, so it's important to pay close attention to what your doctor says at that time.

Most patients can return to modest exercises like walking and easy stretching within two weeks. However, it's imperative to stay away from activities like heavy lifting and vigorous activity that could irritate the nasal passages or throat.

Many patients report feeling almost normal by the end of the third week, with reduced discomfort and better breathing. It's crucial to keep things easy and steer clear of anything that can impede the healing process, though.

Recheck Appointments And Expectations

Your doctor will arrange follow-up appointments after an adenoidectomy to check on your recovery and assess your progress. These consultations are essential for identifying any possible issues early on and taking immediate action.

Your doctor will examine your nose and throat passageways at your follow-up consultations to gauge how well your recovery is going. If necessary, they might also carry out further examinations or imaging studies.

To facilitate your healing process, your doctor might suggest certain lifestyle changes or extra therapies, depending on how well you're recovering individually.

Things Not To Do While Recovering

After an adenoidectomy, it's critical to avoid activities that could aggravate the wound or delay healing during the recovery phase. Among them are:

Exercise That Is Too Hard: It is best to avoid engaging in activities that put a lot of strain on the neck and nasal passages, such as heavy lifting or vigorous physical effort.

Smoking: Smoking irritates the nose and throat passageways, which slows recovery and raises the possibility of problems.

Talking Too Much: Prolonged or loud talking can strain the throat muscles and slow the healing process.

Foods that are spicy or acidic: These might irritate the nasal and throat passages, resulting in pain and delaying the healing process.

Dietary Guidelines Following Surgery

Maintaining a soft, bland diet is crucial after an adenoidectomy to reduce inflammation of the nasal and throat passages. Following surgery, the following food suggestions are:

Soft Foods: Choose foods like soups, yogurt, mashed potatoes, and scrambled eggs that are soft and simple to swallow.

Cold or Room Temperature Foods: Steer clear of hot or cold foods and drinks since these can cause throat irritation.

Hydration: To stay hydrated and maintain a moist throat, consume lots of liquids. Herbal teas, broth, and water are all healthy choices.

Eat Nothing Irritating: Foods that can irritate the throat and nasal passages should be avoided, such as those that are spicy, acidic, or crunchy.

Recognizing And Handling Any Postponed Issues

Although adenoidectomy is typically considered safe, problems might occur during the early phase of healing. It's critical to be aware of these possible side effects and to get help from a doctor if you notice any worrying symptoms. Following an adenoidectomy, some late problems could include:

Persistent discomfort: If your throat discomfort is ongoing or getting worse, it may be a sign of an infection or another underlying problem.

Breathing Problems: Prolonged nasal congestion or breathing problems may be signs of a complication like nasal polyps or the development of scar tissue.

Persistent Bleeding: Although modest bleeding is common in the days after surgery, severe bleeding has to be checked out by a physician.

Sleep problems: Following an adenoidectomy, if you continue to have sleep apnea, snore loudly, or have other sleep problems, you may need to be evaluated and treated further.

Maintaining vigilance and promptly seeking medical assistance in the event of any concerned symptoms can aid in facilitating a seamless and prosperous recuperation following an adenoidectomy.

CHAPTER SEVEN

COMMON ISSUES AND DIFFICULTIES

Despite being a safe and common treatment, adenoidectomy can cause anxiety among patients and caregivers due to possible consequences. Anxiety can be reduced and a quicker healing process can be guaranteed by being aware of these worries and the potential consequences.

After an adenoidectomy, postoperative pain and discomfort are a regular worry. After the treatment, it's common for patients—especially kids—to have sore throats. When the throat heals, this pain usually goes away in a few days. Acetaminophen and ibuprofen are two examples of over-the-counter pain medications that can help control pain and reduce inflammation. In addition, drinking cold liquids or sucking on ice chips might help.

An additional typical postoperative problem is a low-grade fever. In the days after surgery, a little rise in body temperature is normal and typically indicates that the body is fending off an infection. However, it's critical to get in touch with your healthcare professional right away if the fever lasts longer than expected or if it's accompanied by other worrisome symptoms like excruciating pain or trouble breathing.

Handling Typical Postoperative Problems

Taking care of common postoperative problems like fever or sore throats is crucial to a quick recovery. Supporting the body's healing process requires promoting enough sleep and hydration. Staying hydrated and relieving sore throats can be achieved by consuming an ample amount of fluids, including clear broth or water.

Throat lozenges or sprays can reduce soreness and discomfort in addition to relieving pain. But to avoid choking concerns, it is imperative that lozenges not be given to young children. As a calming treat, think about serving ice cream or popsicles instead.

Identifying Infection Or Complication Signs

Even though complications from adenoidectomy are uncommon, it's important to remain watchful and identify any warning indications. Infection symptoms should be treated right away, such as fever that doesn't go away, discomfort that doesn't go better, or foul-smelling discharge from the throat or nose.

Breathing difficulties, heavy bleeding, or signs of dehydration are some other indications of problems. Do not hesitate to get in touch with your healthcare practitioner for additional assessment and advice if your child exhibits any worrisome symptoms or if their condition does not get better as planned.

When to Speak with Your Physician

When it comes to getting timely medical assistance when needed, knowing when to call your doctor is essential. Seek immediate medical attention following an adenoidectomy if you or your kid has significant discomfort, a prolonged fever, difficulty breathing, or any other troubling symptoms.

In the same way, don't be afraid to ask your healthcare practitioner any questions or concerns you may have regarding the healing process or the postoperative care recommendations. They can answer any questions you may have and offer tailored advice based on your unique circumstances.

Resolving The Concerns Of Parents And Caregivers

A parent or caregiver's assistance is essential to a child's rehabilitation after an adenoidectomy. While it's normal to be worried about the operation and its possible side effects, being knowledgeable helps ease worry and gives parents the confidence they need to give their children the care they need.

To address any worries or inquiries parents may have, it is essential to have open communication with healthcare providers. Parents can feel more secure in their abilities to assist their child's recovery if they are informed about the surgery, any dangers, and postoperative care instructions beforehand.

Techniques For A Quick And Problem-Free Recuperation

To maximize the results of an adenoidectomy, techniques for a painless and complication-free recovery must be put into practice. Getting enough sleep, staying hydrated, and managing discomfort are essential components of postoperative care.

Encouragement of a soft diet rich in foods that are easily swallowed can aid in healing and help avoid throat irritation.

Reducing the chance of problems and promoting a quicker recovery can also be achieved by avoiding physically demanding activities and contact with sick people.

Scheduling follow-up sessions with your healthcare practitioner is crucial for tracking your recovery's progress and addressing any issues that may come up.

You can contribute to a favorable outcome after an adenoidectomy by carefully adhering to postoperative care instructions and keeping an eye out for any indications of difficulties.

CHAPTER EIGHT

DETAILED FAQS

An adenoidectomy: what is it? The surgical removal of the adenoids, which are little lumps of tissue at the rear of the nasal cavity, is known as an adenoidectomy. As a component of the immune system, adenoids aid in the defense against infections; nevertheless, they can occasionally expand or develop a persistent infection, which can lead to respiratory troubles, ear infections, or disturbed sleep.

Adenoidectomy: Who needs one? The most frequent candidates for adenoidectomy are children. It is frequently advised in cases where a child has prolonged nasal congestion that doesn't improve with conventional therapies, sleep apnea, recurrent throat or ear infections, or trouble breathing through their nose. If an adult has persistent infections or comparable symptoms, they may require an operation.

How is the process carried out? Under general anesthesia, the procedure is typically performed. There is no need for external incisions because the surgeon accesses the adenoids through the mouth. Using surgical tools or an electrocautery device, the adenoids are removed, and to stop any bleeding, the region is cauterized.

How does the healing process work? Resting at home for a few days is usually necessary for recovery. Over-the-counter pain medications can be used to treat minor pain, discomfort, or sore throats that patients may suffer. It's crucial to adhere to the surgeon's post-operative care recommendations, which include drinking plenty of water and eating soft foods.

Does an adenoidectomy come with any risks? While there is always a chance of problems, major ones are uncommon after surgery. Bleeding, infection, or anesthesia-related adverse responses are examples of potential dangers. The majority of people heal without any major problems.

Frequently Asked Questions About Adenoidectomy Addressed

What is the duration of the surgery? The length of time needed for an adenoidectomy procedure varies based on the patient's age and case complexity, typically lasting between 20 and 45 minutes.

Does it hurt? Patients won't experience any discomfort during the surgery because they are under general anesthesia. Sore throats following surgery are frequent, although they can be treated with painkillers.

When can an adult have an adenoidectomy? Yes, although adenoidectomy is more prevalent in children, adults can still get one if their quality of life is being negatively impacted by recurrent problems.

When is my kid's last day of school? After surgery, most kids can go back to school in about a week. Before allowing them to resume their regular activities, be sure they are comfortable and have fully recovered.

Excerpts From Myths And Misconceptions

Myth: Having an adenoidectomies will impair immunity. Although the adenoids are a component of the immune system, their removal has little effect on the body's capacity to combat infections. The tonsils and lymph nodes, among other immune system components, keep functioning regularly.

Myth: Adenoidectomy is only necessary for children. Although adenoidectomy is a more common treatment in children, adults may also benefit if they have breathing issues or persistent infections because of swollen adenoids.

Myth: The procedure hurts so bad. Patients are not in pain during the treatment because they are under general anesthesia. Typically, post-operative pain is minimal and treatable with medicine.

Testimonials And Experiences From Patients

Jane's Experience: "My daughter was always congested and suffered from ear infections." Her state of health significantly improved following the adenoidectomy. She quickly returned to her playful self after a simple recovery.

Michael's Story: "My persistent sinus infections were excruciating, but even as an adult, I was dubious about needing an adenoidectomy. The healing went more smoothly than I had anticipated after the speedy surgery. I can sleep soundly and breathe easily now.

Advice on Selecting the Best Hospital and Surgeon

Investigate Credentials: Seek a surgeon with a great deal of expertise doing adenoidectomies and board certification in otolaryngology. Examine their qualifications and patient testimonials.

Visit the Facility: Take a look around the clinic or hospital where the surgery is scheduled to be done. Verify its accreditation and track record for patient care and safety.

Ask Questions: During your appointment, enquire about the surgeon's background, the particulars of the operation, and the anticipated results. Having clear communication is essential to being informed and at ease.

A hospital that offers complete post-operative care and assistance, including convenient access to follow-up consultations and emergency services in case of need, is the one you should choose.

Other Sources for More Reading and Assistance

Books and Articles: Adenoidectomy is covered in great length in several enlightening books and articles, which also include the science underlying the treatment and the most recent study results.

Support Groups: Attending an in-person or virtual support group can offer priceless emotional support as well as useful guidance from those who have had the surgery.

Medical Websites: Reputable medical websites with extensive information on adenoidectomy, including patient guides and professional advice, include the Mayo Clinic and WebMD.

Healthcare Providers: If necessary, your pediatrician or primary care physician can refer you to a specialist and offer more information. Please don't be afraid to contact them with any questions or issues you may have.